Disclaimer Notice

Please note the information contained within this document is for educational and entertainment purposes only. Considerable energy and every attempt has been made to provide the most up to date, accurate, relative, reliable, and complete information, but the reader is strongly encouraged to seek professional advice prior to using any of this information contained in this book. The reader understands they are reading and using this information contained herein at their own risk, and in no way will the author, publisher, or any affiliates be held responsible for any damages whatsoever. No warranties of any kind are expressed or implied. Readers acknowledge that the author is not engaging in the rendering of legal, financial, medical, or any other professional advice. By reading this document, the reader agrees that under no circumstances is the author, publisher, or anyone else affiliated with the production, distribution, sale, or any other element of this book responsible for any losses, direct or indirect, which are incurred as a result of the use of information contained within this document, including, but not limited to, -errors, omissions, or inaccuracies. Because of the rate with which conditions change, the author and publisher reserve the right to alter and update the information contained herein on the new conditions whenever they see applicable.

Ultimate Body Butter Recipes Guide!

Body Butter Recipes

50 All Natural Body Butter Recipes To Hydrate, Refresh, And Rejuvenate Your Skin To Look Younger, Healthier And More Naturally Beautiful!

Lilly Sparks

STOP!!! Before you read any further....Would you like to know the secrets of Anti Ageing?

If your answer is yes, then you are not alone. Thousands of people are looking for the secret to reducing wrinkles, looking younger, and maintaining a youthful appearance.

If you have been searching for these answers without much luck, you are in the right place!

Not only will you gain incredible insight in this book, but because I want to make sure to give you as much value as possible, right now for a limited time you can get full **100% FREE access to a VIP bonus Ebook** entitled **Anti Ageing Made Easy!**

Just Go Here For Free Instant Access:

www.LuxyLifeNaturals.com

Table Of Contents

Introduction

I want to thank you and congratulate you for purchasing the book, "Body Butter Recipes".

This "Body Butter Recipes" book contains proven steps and strategies on how to create effective body butters.

Body butteris slightly different from lotion because it has a thicker consistency. It has intense moisturizing benefits and is ideal to use for dry and rough skin. Commercial body butters are filled with chemicals and synthetic ingredients that can seep into your pores and cause damage into your body system. Making your own body butter allows you to control the ingredients and personalize it according to your needs and preference.

This book also contains information on other body products like soap and organic lotion. Using these homemade natural products can provide a lot of benefit for your skin and overall wellbeing.

Thanks again for purchasing this book. I hope you enjoy it!

Chapter 1: Look Younger By Taking Care Of Your Skin

The skin is the largest organ of the body. It keeps foreign elements from entering the internal system. The human skin is always growing where the old cells dying and new cells are forming.

Healthy skin is also an indication of good health. If you are suffering from disease and illness, you skin can became pale and dull. Proper skin care is essential if you want to look younger.

Eat for your skin

Your diet can greatly affect your skin;a healthy and balanced diet in particular can give you a youthful glow. Foods high in omega 3 fatty acid can help regenerate your skin. Antioxidants can protect the skin from free radical damage. Vitamin E rich foods also help you skin glow.

Stay hydrated

Water is essential to maintain the proper function of the body. Consuming enough water can keep your skin supple. Dehydrated skin looks rough and can promote wrinkles.

Proper skin care

You do not need expensive creams or elaborate skin rituals to look young. Just remember to cleanse, ex-foliate and moisturize your skin on a regular basis to maintain its youthful glow. Wash your skin with a gently cleanser to remove dirt, make-up and debris. Ex-foliate your skin with a scrub 1-3 times in a week. This helps remove dead skin cell build-up and promote faster skin cell turnover. Do not forget to apply lotion and moisturizer. Aging skin can dry quickly so you have to replenish the moisture.

Homemade skin care

Although there are products for almost all skin problems, you can also choose to create your own skin products. Aside from being more economical, making your own products can help you control the ingredients in it.

Chapter 2: Benefits Of Homemade Body Butter

Body butters are thick creams that can hydrate the skin. You can use a lot of ingredients for your homemade body butter. Making your own body butter also has a lot of advantages.

Safe to Use

The skin tends to absorb anything that you apply. Commercial body butters contain chemicals and ingredients that can be harmful to your health. Natural and homemade body butter does not contain toxic ingredients and only contain natural oil from nuts and seeds.

Offers Protection

Body butter can form a barrier of protection which can protect the skin from environmental pollutants.

Nourishes the Skin

Body butters are rich in omega 3 fatty acid that can moisturize the skin and reduce inflammation. Body butter also contains vitamins like vitamin C and E which are powerful antioxidants.

Softer Skin

Regularly applying body butter can make your skin silky soft. You can easily eliminate dry and cracked skin by using body butter.

Affordable

You may need to invest in essential equipment and ingredients but you will save money in the long run by making your own body butter. You can also make several batches and give it away as gifts.

Versatile

Body butters may be mainly used to moisturize the skin but it can also be used for different purposes. You can use it as an aftershave or as a makeup remover. You can also apply body butter in your cuticles to soften it. It can also be used as an alternative to oil in massage therapy.

Chapter 3: Why Should You Switch To An Organic Lotion?

Regularly applying lotion can make your skin feeling soft. It also promotes healthier skin regeneration. Lotion has a thinner consistency compared to body butter. It is ideal to use during the summer when you sweat a lot or if you have a very oily skin.

Safe and Natural Ingredients

The main benefit of using organic lotion is its ingredients. Organic lotion does not contain chemicals and toxins that can harm your health.

Absorbs Easily

Organic lotion can make your skin soft for a long period of time. Since it does not contain any synthetic ingredients, the lotion gets absorbed into the skin easier. Commercial lotions contain chemicals that sit on top of the skin and can make it look oily.

Paraben free

Paraben are synthetic ingredients that act like a preservative. They interfere with the natural function of the endocrine system. Organic products do not contain parabens.

No Artificial Fragrance

Lotions are known for their fragrance. However, artificial fragrance is used to mask the odor of chemicals. Strong fragrances can also cause headaches and allergy for some people. It is better to choose lotions that contain natural fragrances like essential oil.

Good for Sensitive Skin

People suffering from sensitive skin can benefit from using organic lotion since it is milder to the skin and does not trigger irritation.

Environmentally Friendly

Organic lotions are more environmentally friendly since no toxic, synthetic chemicals are added in the process of creating it.

Chapter 4: Natural Soap Making For Beginners

Soap is an essential product to clean the skin. Just like body butters and lotions, you can also benefit from using homemade soaps made with natural ingredients. There are different processes in making soap:

Melt and Pour

The melt and pour method of soap making is recommended for beginners since it is easy to do and you don't have to handle lye directly. You will need to purchase a clear bar of glycerine soap and melt it in a pot. You can then add essential oils, herbs or any infusion that you want. Pour the mixture in a mold and let it solidify.

Cold Process

Cold pressed soap is made from fatty acids and lye. The fatty acid can come from plant or animal fat like beef tallow and coconut oil. Cold process soap making can be considered as an art and science. The water, fat and lye create a chemical reaction known as saponification that creates the soap. The process can take up to six weeks to complete.

You have to be careful when creating cold pressed soap since the lye can be dangerous to handle. You may need to use goggles and gloves to protect yourself.

Hot Process

Hot process soap is a great take on the cold process soap method. In a nutshell, you will combine all your ingredients in a pot and heat it until it completely melts. The water evaporates and the mixture is poured into a mold, and then cooled.

Chapter 5: Sample Recipes Of Soap Making For Beginners

You create natural soaps using different soap methods. Aside from being practical and efficient, making your own soap can also be fun.

Oatmeal Soap (Melt and Pour Method)

8 oz clear glycerin soap

40 drops of sweet almond oil

½ cup rolled oats

Instructions:

Cut the clear soap into cubes then place it in a bowl. Melt the clear soap in the microwave for about 2-3 minutes. Add the sweet almond oil extract. Stir to combine. Place the oatmeal in a food processor then blend until the grains become smaller. Add the rolled oatmeal to the soap. Stir and then pour into your desired mold. Let it solidify before using.

Honey Beeswax Soap (Cold Process Method)

0.55 oz cocoa butter

2.75 olive oil

1.1 oz sunflower seed oil

3.6 oz distilled water

0.8 oz honey

3.3 oz coconut oil

3.3 oz palm oil

1.6 oz lye

1 tsp sodium lactate

Instructions:

Make sure that you work in a well ventilated area. Gently pour the lye into the water. Stir the mixture until clear. Mix in the sunflower oil and olive oil. Stir to combine. Once the water and lye are about 120 degrees, pour it to the oils. Whisk the mixture using a stick blender until it has a light trace. Add the honey and blend again. Pour the soap into your desired mold and let it age for 5 days before removing from the mold.

Apple Spice Soap (Hot Process Method)

8 oz coconut oil

12 oz distilled water

1 tbsp apple spice

2 tbsp apple essential oil

18 oz canola oil

18 oz olive oil

6 oz lye

1 tbsp turmeric

Instructions:

Set your oven at 200 degrees. Pour the lye on the water. Let it cool until the mixture reaches 100 degrees. Melt the oil and let it cool.

Combine the lye water and oil. Whisk using a blender. Add the apple spice and essential oil. Place the mixture in the oven for 1 ½ hours. Pour in a mold. Wait for 24 hours before removing from the mold.

Chapter 6: TheBenefits OfCoconut Oil On Your Skin

Coconut oil is famous all over the world as a versatile ingredient. It can be used on the skin or added into food.

Coconut Oil Composition

Coconut oil is predominantly composed of saturated fats. It keeps the skin soft and smooth. It also retains the moisture in the skin and prevents drying.

Coconut oil has great antimicrobial properties that can protect the skin from infection and germs. This benefit can also be experienced if the coconut oil is ingested. Coconut oil contains lauric acid that can break the fatty acids easily which can be transformed to usable energy quickly.

Coconut oil also contains vitamin E that can help repair the skin cells and protect the skin from cracking. It has great anti aging properties that prevents premature aging. The best benefit of coconut oil is that it does not become rancid unlike other oils. You can store and use it for a longer period of time.

Uses of Coconut Oil for Skin

Skin softener

Natural lotions and body butters usually contain coconut oil. It can help relieve dry and cracked skin. Coconut oil is also great to use for hard and cracked skin and can sooth your tired feet. It is also great to add to your natural scrubs because it can help in skin regeneration. You can remove skin impurities without leaving the skin irritated.

Make-up Remover

Coconut oil is a cheap and effective make-up remover. It does not contain chemicals so you do not have to worry about it getting into your eyes and delicate areas.

Skin problems

Coconut oil has been proven to be effective for many skin disorders like acne, eczema and psoriasis. Much of its benefits come from its protein content which can replace old skin cells with new. Its antibacterial properties can also heal skin disorders without any side effect.

Chapter 7: Using Essential Oil

Essential oils have been used for thousands of years for cosmetic, spiritual and health purposes. The oil is extracted through distillation or cold processing to ensure that the oil is in its purest form.

Inspire Positivity

Each essential oil has its own characteristics and unique composition. Each types of oil has a different effect on your emotional state. For example, orange essential oil can be invigorating while lavender oil has calming effects.

Enhance your physical wellness

Essential oils can help improve your physical well being. It is usually added to homemade products like lotion to boosts its benefits. Essential oils can also replace chemicals in your skin products. Essential oils can promote clear, supple and healthy skin.

Create spiritual awareness

Essential oils have been used for thousands of years in religious and spiritual ceremonies. People believed that these oils can help a person connect to something that is larger than himself. The scent of oils can stimulate olfactory receptor in the brain that is associated with memory and emotion.

Chapter 8: How To Use Body Butter For Anti-Aging

Body butter has become really popular because of its amazing benefits. There are a lot of ingredients that you can use depending on your needs and personal preference.

How to Use Body Butter

Body butter is best applied after taking a warm shower to moisturize your skin. The main difference between body butter and lotion is their consistency. Body butter is thicker than lotion. Body butters are very moisturizing on the skin and can help relieve dry and cracked skin.

You need to apply the butter all over your body including hard reaching areas like the back and legs. Focus on wrinkled body parts like the knees, elbows and feet. Since body butter are great for scars and stretch marks, be sure to apply it on those areas as well.

Common Body Butter Ingredients with Anti-aging Properties

Almond Oil

It contains Vitamin B1, B2, B6, A and E. It also promotes a healthy skin glow.

Coconut Oil

It is great for hydrating dry skin. It can also protect the skin from sunburn and prevents wrinkles.

Shea Butter

It is a rich source of fatty acids and vitamins that can enhance collagen formation.

Jojoba Oil

It has anti-inflammatory and antibacterial properties that can treat skin conditions and help make the skin look fresh and young.

Chapter 9: Body Butter Recipes

A good skin care routine includes applying moisturizer and body butter to prevent dryness and to protect the skin from environmental damage. Making your own body butter is an economical and fun way to manage your skin without having to purchase expensive creams. You can easily personalize your body butter and include your favorite ingredients.

Body Butter Making Steps:

Choose a foundation

The most common base of body butters is organic beeswax. Make sure that you get pure beeswax for best results. Most suppliers sell their beeswax in blocks. You can keep the extra ingredients for future body butter creations.

Some recipes do not include beeswax. Instead, it incorporates fats like coconut oil, Shea butter, mango butter and cocoa butter.

Add Oils

Once you have your base, you can add any ingredient to create a beautiful blend that can fit your needs. Make sure that you do not have any allergy to any of the ingredients that you are going to use. You can do a skin test first before adding it to your body butter.

Mix the ingredients

Melt the beeswax in a double broiler method. This is where you set a metal or heat-proof glass bowl on a pot of boiling water. Stir the beeswax until it is fully melted. Add plant or animal oils like coconut oil, shea oil, beef tallow or cocoa butter next. Stir the mixture until completely melted. Add the essential oil and other ingredients. Let it cool. You have the option of whipping your body butter to make it lighter. Pour the mixture into your desired container.

Storing your body butters

Body butter can solidify at room temperature. You can pour it in silicon molds or store them into containers with lids to prevent them from drying out.

Chapter 10: 50 All Natural Body Butter Recipes

The recipes in this chapter have the same procedure. Make sure that you follow the body butter making steps in the previous chapter.

1. Lavender Body Butter

Lavender body butter is great for relaxing and rejuvenating the skin.

4 tbsp coconut oil

2 tbsp beeswax

3 tbsp aloe vera gel

10 drops lavender essential oil

1 ½ tbsp olive oil

2 tbsp honey

2 tsp lanolin

1 vitamin E capsule

2. Mango Citrus Body Butter

Citrus fragrances can energize you and invigorate your senses. The mango butter adds a fruity fragrance.

25 g cocoa butter

25 g mango butter

1 tsp vitamin E

10 g beeswax

30 g shea butter

1 tsp almond oil

20 drops citrus essential oil

3. Magnesium Body Butter

Magnesium can sooth your skin and leave is silky smooth.

½ cup magnesium flakes

¼ cup unrefined coconut oil

3 tbsp Shea butter

2 tbsp beeswax

Note: Melt the magnesium flaxes in 3 tbsp of boiling water before adding to the other melted ingredients.

4. Rosemary Mint Whipped Shea Butter

This is a luxurious body butter that provides long lasting moisture and skin protection.

45 g cocoa butter

45 g kukui nut oil

10 drops rosemary essential oil

90 g Shea butter

20 drops spearmint essential oil

5. Coconut Rose Body Butter

This is a great body butter that can retain natural moisture in the skin. The rose essential oil adds anti aging benefits to the body butter.

10 g jojoba oil

3 g cornstarch

60 g refined coconut oil

1 ml alkanet infused oil

10 drops rose essential oil

Note: Wait until the butter is cooled at room temperature before adding the rose essential oil.

6. Glowing Skin Body Butter

Make your skin glow by using natural plant oil like coconut oil and Shea butter.

2 cups extra virgin coconut oil

1 drop tea tree oil

10 drops jasmine oil

7 oz Shea butter

7. Sacred Frankincense Whipped Body Butter

Frankincense was used in religious ceremonies and practices. It has a musky and earthy fragrance.

½ cup organic virgin coconut oil

½ cup mango butter

1 tsp vitamin E oil

½ cup Shea butter

1 oz raw organic cocoa butter

30 drops sacred frankincense essential oil

8. Wild Orange Body Butter

This is a great body butter recipe that is perfect for beginners. This body butter has moisturizing property and can also help heal scars because of its vitamin E content.

1 cup cocoa butter

8 drops vitamin E oil

2 tbsp almond oil

8 drops wild orange oil

9. Edible Chocolate Body Butter

You can make your body butter and eat it too! Turn chocolate into sensual body butter. Make sure to keep this at room temperature.

¾ cup coconut oil, melted

½ tbsp vanilla powder

1/3 cup agave nectar

¼ cup cacao powder

Optional Add-ons

1 tspmaca

½ tspcistanche

10. Cinnamon Body Butter

Cinnamon also has strong antibacterial and anti fungal properties. It has astringent components similar to witch hazel. It can reduce inflammation and cellulite.

100 g coconut oil

50 grams Shea butter

Cinnamon stick, blend until it is reduced to small pieces

50 g cocoa butter

30 drops cinnamon oil

11. Peppermint Body Butter

Peppermint body butter is a luxurious skin moisturizer that is great to give as a gift during the holidays.

6 oz coconut oil

20 drops peppermint oil

2 oz cocoa butter

12. Soothing Body Butter

You can use this as a shaving cream. It can lessen the risk of getting ingrown hair and acts as a gentle deodorant.

½ cup coconut oil

2 tbsp jojoba oil

20 drops of tea tree oil

6 tbsp cocoa butter

13. Coffee Butter

Apply this skin to your tired skin for an indulgent treat. Coffee is a natural stimulant that can instantly perk you up.

0.7 oz white beeswax

2.4 oz sunflower oil

1 oz emulsifying wax

5 ml dark rich chocolate fragrance oil

0.2 oz grapefruit seed extract

3.1 oz coffee butter

1.2 ozstearic acid

15.6 oz distilled water

5 ml peppermint essential oil

14. Vanilla Bean Body Butter

The vanilla bean body butter is easy to make and has a rich and sensual fragrance.

½ cup sweet almond oil

1 vanilla bean

1 cup raw cocoa butter

½ cup coconut oil

Note: Process the vanilla bean in a food processor or coffee grinder before using.

15. Lemon Cream Body Butter

Moisturizing body butter is great to use during the winter. This recipe has no beeswax so it melts easily when applied to skin.

6 tbsp coconut oil

1 tbsp vitamin E oil

¼ cup cacao butter

¼ tsp lemon essential oil

16. Luxurious Body Butter

You can also use rose petals and rosemary to create your body butter. This is a great option if you do not have essential oils at hand.

2 tbsp Shea butter

1 tbsp olive oil

1 ml vitamin E oil

1 tbsp mint infused coconut oil

1 cup dried rose petals

2 tbsp fresh rosemary

Note: Add the rose petals and rosemary in a pot of boiling water. Strain the liquid and add to the other ingredients.

17. Plum Whipped Body Butter

This body butter looks very feminine with its light pink color and sweet fragrance.

2 oz organic virgin coconut cream oil

1 oz plum kernel oil

1 ½ tsp plum jojoba wax beads

2 ozultra refined cocoa butter

½ oz carnauba wax

18. Blissful Body Butter

Shea butter is a common ingredient in many homemade body butters. It is naturally moisturizing and also has a delicious fragrance. The vanilla, ylangylang and bergamot combine well to create a wonderful aroma.

3 oz peach kernel oil

1 oz jojoba oil

5 oz Shea butter

3 oz safflower oil

1 tsp cornstarch

For the essential oil blend:

25 drops bergamot essential oil

15 drops vanilla oil

5 drops ylangylang

19. Bronzing Body Butter

This body butter can give your skin a sun kissed glow. It is perfect to use during the winter to avoid looking pale. This body butter will not stain your clothes.

1 cup Shea butter

½ cup olive oil

1 tsp natural vitamin E oil

½ cup coconut oil

2 tbsp cocoa powder

10 drops essential oil of choice

Note: Make sure to label the body butter since it can look and smell like chocolate and children might accidentally eat it.

20. Green Tea Body Butter

Green tea is known for its therapeutic and health benefits. It has great antioxidant properties that can protect the skin form damage.

2.5 oz beeswax

2 ozshea butter

1 tbspmatcha

2 oz mango butter

1 oz almond butter

1 tbsp coconut oil

21. Cranberry Body Butter

Cranberries can fight free radicals and keeps your skin fresh. It also adds a delicate pink hue to your body butter.

¼ cup coconut oil

1 tbsp frozen cranberries

1 tbspShea butter

1 drop orange essential oil

22. Beach Body Butter

This cream can make your skin buttery smooth. It is great to use after a day at the beach to replenish the moisture of the skin.

2 oz cocoa butter

2 ozmonoi butter

3 tsp sweet almond oil

¼ tsp vitamin E oil

2 oz Shea butter

1 tspargan oil

3 tsp aloe vera oil

3 tsp coconut oil

23. Simple Coconut and Vanilla Body Butter

This is a great party favor for women. You can give it away during your wedding or baby shower. It is simple and easy to create to make and cost less than other body butters so you can create a larger batch.

3 cups coconut oil

3 tbsp vanilla extract

Note: You do not need to melt the coconut oil thoroughly. Just whisk it and add the vanilla extract.

24. Lavender Body Butter Bars

Body butter bars function like a regular skin moisturizer but it contains more beeswax so it can solidify into bars. To use, simple rub it in your skin. The natural heat from the body will melt the butter and make it easier to apply.

2 oz beeswax

2 oz Shea butter

2 oz coconut oil

20 drops lavender essential oil

Note: Make sure to give it a few hours to set. Remember that extreme hot temperatures can still melt body butter bars.

25. Raspberry Truffle Bars

This is perfect for a valentine treat. The raspberry and passion flower have a romantic aroma. Pour it in a heart shaped mold to make it more appropriate.

1 ½ oz beeswax

4 oz cocoa butter

1 oz red raspberry seed oil

¼ oz raspberry truffle oil

1 tsp red jojoba wax beads

2 ozbabassu oil

¼ oz passion flower oil

26. Margarita Body Cream

35 g organic lemon balm hydrosol

2 g glycerin

35 g water

3 g grapefruit extract

12 g mango butter

12 g peach kernel oil

2 g stearic acid

12 g cocoa butter

10 g emulsifying wax

1 tbsp parsley powder

Note: Heat the first four ingredients in a separate double broiler before adding to the remaining ingredients. Keep refrigerated.

27. Blossoms Body Cream

The aromatic essential oils for this butter give it a potent floral scent.

12 g mango butter

12 g babassu butter

3 g grapefruit extract

12 g cocoa butter

10 g emulsifying wax

15 drops bergamot oil

10 drops lavender oil

10 drops ylangylang oil

28. Rain forest Flower Body Cream

This is a thick body butter cream that has intense moisturizing properties.

7 g cocoa butter

7 g maracuja oil

5 g beeswax

7 g andiroba oil

7 g jojoba

10 drops carrot seed extract

10 drops bergamot oil

10 drops arnica extract

29. Eczema Relief Body Butter

The coconut oil, vitamin E and oatmeal can provide relief for eczema.

1 cup olive oil

2 tbsp vitamin E oil

1 cup coconut oil

½ cup beeswax

¼ cup ground oatmeal, finely ground

30. Coffee Bean Toning Body Butter

Coffee can reduce the appearance of cellulite and helps you look more toned.

4 oz coffee infused oil

20 drops lemon grass essential oil

20 drops rose geranium essential oil

4 oz cocoa butter

31. Orange Chocolate Poppy Seeds Body Butter

1 tbsp cocoa powder

1 tbsp poppy seeds

4 oz cocoa butter

40 drops sweet orange oil

Note: Boil a cup of water and add the poppy seeds. Strain it and then add the liquid to the ingredients.

32. Chocolate Mint Body Butter

Chocolate and mint is not only a great combination for food; it also smells great when applied on the skin.

1 ozShea butter

1 tbsp cocoa powder

2 oz cocoa butter

1 oz olive butter

20 drop peppermint essential oil

33. Bug Repellent Body Butter Bars

Protect your family from insect bites with this moisturizing body butter bar. You can make smaller bars for your children and place it in a portable container.

¼ cup coconut oil

¼ cup grated beeswax

¼ tsp purification oil blended

¼ cup cocoa butter

¼ tsp vitamin E oil

¼ tsp Thieves oil blend

34. Non-toxic Sunscreen Body Butter Bars

Commercial sunscreen contains chemicals and ingredients that can seep into your blood stream.

½ cup Shea butter

½ cup coconut oil

½ tsp vitamin E oil

5 tbsp beeswax

2 tbsp zinc oxide

¾ tsp lavender oil

Note: Add the zinc oxide last before you pour it into your desired mold.

35. Whipped Gingerbread Body Butter

Gingerbread is a popular scent during the winter. This body butter makes your skin supple, smooth and glowing.

½ cup Shea butter

2 tbsp almond oil

2 tsp ground ginger

1 tsp vanilla extract

¼ cup coconut oil

2 tsp vitamin E

1 tsp ground cinnamon

36. **Whipped Jasmine Tallow** Body Butter

Tallow is an animal fat that closely resembles the cellular composition of humans. Tallow is also easily absorbed by the skin.

1 cup Shea butter

½ cup jojoba oil

2 tsp vitamin E oil

½ cup tallow

1 tsp jasmine essential oil

37. **Peppermint Cinnamon Body Butter**

This body butter combination is perfect for Christmas. It has the perfect blend of cinnamon, chocolate, almond and peppermint.

1 ½ tbsp cocoa butter

2 tbsp coconut oil

¼ tsp vegetable glycerin

20 drops peppermint essential oil

1 ½ tbsp beeswax

2 tbsp almond oil

4 drops vitamin E oil

12 drops cinnamon essential oil

1 tbsp zinc oxide

38.Pumpkin Pie Spice Body Butter

This is a rich body butter that can easily replace your commercial skin moisturizer. The pumpkin spice scent is perfect for fall. You do not need to refrigerate this body butter since the vitamin E acts as a natural preservative.

½ cup Shea butter

2 tbsp olive oil

3 tsp pumpkin pie spice

¼ cup coconut oil

2 vitamin E oil

1 tsp vanilla extract

39.Mint and Green Tea Body Butter

A little goes a long way when it comes to body butter. This body butter is easy to make but you may need to place it in the refrigerator for 1 ½ hours to set.

1/3 cup Sea butter

1 tsp olive oil

½ tbspmacha powder

4 drops peppermint oil

½ cup coconut oil

7 drops vitamin E oil

8 mint leaves, finely chopped

Note: Refrigerate and whip the mixture before adding the essential oil and vitamin E.

40. Shea and Coconut Body Butter

Shea and coconut oil have great antibacterial and moisturizing properties. This is one of the simplest body butter recipes.

½ cup Shea butter

¼ cup almond oil

¼ cup coconut oil

41. Rosemary Tea Tree Body Butter

Herbs have therapeutic benefits that can revitalize the skin.

¼ cup coconut oil

10 drops rosemary essential oil

6 tbsp Shea butter

¼ cup almond oil

8 drops tea tree oil

42. All-in One Body Butter

This body butter is very gentle and can even be used on baby's skin

¼ cup cocoa butter

2 tbsp olive oil

¼ tsp Shea butter

1 tbsp castor oil

15 drops chamomile oil

43. Cucumber Body Butter

Cucumber has a soothing and rejuvenating property that can benefit sunburned skin.

4 tbsp fresh cucumber juice oil

5 tbsp coconut oil

2 tbsp almond oil

15 tbsp beeswax

4 tbsp Shea butter

44. Aloe Vera and Coconut Oil Body Butter

Aloe vera is known for its healing properties. This is great to use for scars and stretch marks.

10 drops lavender essential oil

½ cup aloe vera gel

10 drops peppermint essential oil

1 cup coconut oil

45. Pumpkin Body Butter

You can create body butter with your extra pumpkin puree. It is rich in beta carotene which can nourish your skin.

½ cup coconut milk

½ cup pumpkin puree

½ tsp ground cinnamon

46. Ginger and Honey Body Butter

This is a light body butter that is easily absorbed by the skin. It has a sweet and spicy scent from the ginger.

8 g virgin coconut oil

70 g water

2 g raw honey

1 pinch allantoin

7 g emulsifying wax

10 g safflower oil

3 g glycerin

1 pinch silk peptides

47. Dandelion Body Butter Bars

This is great to use for calloused and tired hand. Make sure that you use dandelions that are not sprayed with chemicals. Let the flower dry for a day before infusing it in oil.

1 cup beeswax

1 cup dandelion infused oil

1 cup mango butter

48. Rose Body Butter

Rose is famous for its aesthetic and therapeutic value. Gather rose petals and place them in a jar of olive or sunflower oil. Set it aside for a few days before using.

3 oz rose petal infused oil

15 g beeswax

15 g rosehip oil

49. Good Morning Body Butter

This body butter can gently energize you

2 drops lavender oil

15 drops grapefruit oil

¼ cup beeswax

½ cup water

1 tsp vegetable glycerin

½ cup grape seed oil

1 tbspshea butter

50. Exotic Evening Body Butter

The combination of sandalwood and jasmine provides a romantic and exotic scent.

5 drops sandalwood oil

8 drops jasmine oil

3 drop lime oil

¼ cup beeswax

½ cup coconut oil

½ cup mango butter

Conclusion

Thank you again for purchasing this book on natural body butter!

I am extremely excited to pass this information along to you, and I am so happy that you now have read and can hopefully implement these strategies going forward.

I hope this book was able to help you understand how to create great body products and how to use natural ingredients.

The next step is to get started using this information and to hopefully live a happy and healthy life!

Please don't be someone who just reads this information and doesn't apply it, the strategies in this book will only benefit you if you use them!

If you know of anyone else that could benefit from the information presented here please inform them of this book.

Finally, if you enjoyed this book and feel it has added value to your life in any way, please take the time to share your thoughts and post a review on Amazon. It'd be greatly appreciated!

Thank you and good luck!

Preview Of:

<u>Minimalism</u>

Discover Minimalism, Declutter, And Be Stress Free Living The Lifestyle Of Simplicity In 10 Easy Steps!

Introduction

I want to thank you and congratulate you for purchasing the book, "Minimalism: Discover Minimalism, Declutter, And Be Stress Free Living The Lifestyle Of Simplicity In 10 Easy Steps!".

This "Minimalism" book contains proven steps and strategies on how to apply the principle of minimalism in your life so that you can have a happy and meaningful life that is devoid of distractions and stress.

Minimalism entails a person to live only with the barest necessities so that he may ultimately focus on those things that he truly enjoys. For someone who is utterly consumed by material things and is drowned by a hectic lifestyle, embracing minimalism is definitely a daunting task. As such, this book is here to help you transform each day of your life from chaos into peace.

The book consists of ten chapters, which basically will answer these three fundamental questions about minimalism:

- What is minimalism?
- How can you be a minimalist?
- Can you sustain a minimalist lifestyle?

Upon unraveling the answers to these three key questions, hopefully this book can help you transform your life into a clutter-free and stress-free one by just following ten easy steps towards a minimalistic life.

Thanks again for purchasing this book, I hope you enjoy it!

Chapter 1: Reasons Behind Living A Minimalist Lifestyle

Consumerism has become entwined in everyone's lives. As you open your television for the first time during the day, after every segment of your favorite morning show you are exposed to ads about products that claim you need them, when in fact you have lived your whole life just fine without them. As you get into your car and head for work, you are still bombarded by ads – on the sidewalks, in billboards, and in posters. Advertisements are everywhere.

Ads Convert your Wants to Needs

As a consumer, for every single thing that you have, you want it to be the best. You want to achieve perfection in every way, such as having fashionable outfit, getting the trendy shoes and bags, or buying the latest gadgets. That's why advertisements lure you into buying their products through these fantasies of yours. As an example, look at these tag-lines and see if you aren't caught up with these brands until now.

KFC: It's finger lickin' good!

Mac Pro: Beauty outside. Beast inside.

Survivor: Outwit. Outplay. Outlast.

Disneyland: The happiest place on earth.

M&M's: Melts in your mouth, not in your hands.

Along with their catchy tag lines, these brands are big spenders in marketing just to promote their products. Apple, for instance, enhances the aesthetics of their stores to entice people to come in and try their stuff. Even without a commercial, M&M's play into your imaginations through their tag line "melts in your mouth, not in your hands". All of these advertisements are created so that you will think that the product or service that a company is selling is a "need" rather than a "want".

You're Stressed on the Excesses in Your Life

Now, try to search inside of your home for any items that you may not have used for the past month. The mere idea of having items you do not use frequently is a sign that you may be accumulating things that are way past your necessity.

That's the main reason why people these days are more stressed than ever. They take in excessive things in their life. The more stuff you have, the lesser space there is in your house and more things you have to clean. In your daily lives in your home, school, or work, more work for you each day meant less time for breaks and more stress on your part.

These are the very reasons on why minimalism should become relevant for everyone. Minimalism removes these excesses in life so that one can live simply and happy.

Thanks For Previewing My Exciting Book Entitled:

"Minimalism: Discover Minimalism, Declutter, And Be Stress Free Living The Lifestyle Of Simplicity In 10 Easy Steps!"

To purchase this book, simply go to the Amazon Kindle store and simply search:

"MINIMALISM"

Then just scroll down until you see my book. You will know it is mine because you will see my name "Lilly Sparks" underneath the title.

Alternatively, you can visit my author page on Amazon to see this book and other work I have done. Thanks so much, and please don't forget your free bonuses

DON'T LEAVE YET! - CHECK OUT YOUR FREE BONUS BELOW!

Free Bonus Offer: Get Free Access To The www.LuxyLifeNaturals.com VIP Newsletter!

Once you enter your email address you will immediately get free access to this awesome newsletter!

But wait, right now if you join now for free you will also get free access the "Secrets of Becoming A Meditation Expert – In 7 Days!" free Ebook!

To claim both your FREE VIP NEWSLETTER MEMBERSHIP and your FREE BONUS Ebook on the SECRETS OF BECOMING A MEDITATION EXPERT IN 7 DAYS!

Just Go To:

www.LuxyLifeNaturals.com